Depress__

101 Powerful Ways To Beat Depression, Stress, Anxiety And Be Happy

NATURALLY!

New and Improved – 2nd Edition

Shining Universe Energy Books

Table of Contents –

The information provided herein is stated to be truthful and consistent, in that any liability, in terms of inattention or otherwise, by any usage or abuse of any policies, processes, or directions contained within is the solitary and utter responsibility of the recipient reader. Under no circumstances will any legal responsibility or blame be held against the publisher for any reparation, damages, or monetary loss due to the information herein, either directly or indirectly.

Respective authors own all copyrights not held by the publisher.

The information herein is offered for informational purposes solely, and is universal as so. The presentation of the information is without contract or any type of guarantee assurance.

The trademarks that are used are without any consent, and the publication of the trademark is without permission or backing by the trademark owner. All trademarks and brands within this book are for clarifying purposes only and are the owned by the owners themselves, not affiliated with this document.

Introduction

We want to thank you and congratulate you for getting our book, "Depression: 101 powerful ways to beat depression, stress, anxiety and be happy NATURALLY!"

This book contains actionable strategies on how to beat depression and be happy always. The steps mentioned in this book are extremely simple but very powerful and when practiced over a period of time can really make a difference to one's life and overall personality.

Depression affects millions of people worldwide. In fact, it is as common as 'common cold'. Recognizing the problem is the first step but unfortunately, many a times, people do not even realize that they are going through depression.

This book will educate you on how to identify the problem and then show you simple yet powerful techniques of finding a way out of the problem.

Additionally, regular practice of the techniques mentioned in this book will ensure that there is no relapse as well.

Lastly, this book is not just for people suffering from depression but for everyone who want to live a happier healthier life ensuring depression never touches them.

Thank you again for buying this book. We really hope you get immense value from all the efforts put in by us in bringing you this book.

Chapter 1: What Is Depression?

Depression is simply a mood disorder that results in persistent feelings of sadness and helplessness. In other words, depression affects your body, your thoughts, your mood and ordinary habits. Thus, if you are depressed, you experience both physical and emotional problems that could easily make it hard for you to attend to your daily routine just because you don't feel motivated. For instance, you can lose your appetite, have poor sleeping patterns, have low self-esteem and experience a constant feeling of guilt. Additionally, it changes how you behave and how you think. Things that may once have been enjoyable and exciting no longer elicit the same emotions.

Most people have a perception that when you are depressed you are just depressed, not knowing that there are actually different types of depression. For instance, there is postpartum depression that affects women after they give birth. There is also seasonal affective disorder that you are likely to suffer at the onset of winter when there is less natural sunlight. You may also come across psychotic depression where the depression symptoms are so severe that you even hallucinate. These are some of the common types of depression.

Having knowledge of the various kinds of depression gives you an upper hand in knowing how best to deal with depression.

In the following chapter, we will look at how to identify depression and its various symptoms.

Chapter 2: How To Identify The Problem Of Depression

Does it mean that every time you can't manage a smile you are depressed? It definitely does not because there are times when you will be sad and others when you will be happy. So how can you tell you are depressed? In most cases, before you are actually depressed, you will be stressed. Suffering from chronic stress can lead to high levels of cortisol (the stress hormone) and low levels of serotonin and other important neurotransmitters in the brain like dopamine. Consistent high levels of cortisol and low levels of important chemicals can then lead to depression in susceptible people. Therefore, in most cases, if you are stressed for prolonged periods, you are likely to be depressed.

Depression symptoms vary from one person to another, but there are some common signs and symptoms of the disorder. Such symptoms include feelings of hopelessness, followed by overwhelming sadness and helplessness, which, when not addressed, can lead to suicidal thoughts. If you detect a majority of the following signs and symptoms, and they become consistent, it could be a warning that you have depression.

Anger/irritability

You feel restless, agitated or even violent. You develop a short temper, a low tolerance level and everyone and everything gets on your nerves.

Lack of Concentration

Depression causes mental retardation, which results in an inability to process information. This can impair your concentration, making it harder to remember things or make decisions and to focus on ordinary, day-to-day activities. These symptoms can have a negative impact on your thinking process and soon may fill your mind with negative thoughts.

Sleep problems

Changes in sleep patterns range from lack of sleep, referred to as insomnia, to sleeping too much. Other times, you might wake up too early in the morning or have episodes where you wake up several times in a night, say every two or three hours.

Lost interest in daily activities

You become disinterested in activities you previously deemed exciting such as former hobbies, sex, social activities, and pastimes. You have lost your ability to feel pleasure and joy.

Self-loathing

You experience strong feelings of guilt or worthlessness, and harshly criticize yourself for perceived mistakes and faults. You also feel like your entire life is in ruins and, to make matters worse, there is nothing you can do to improve the situation.

Reckless behaviour

Common improper or escapist behaviors may range from reckless driving to compulsive gambling, undertaking dangerous sports, and substance abuse.

Weight changes

You'll notice significant weight gain or weight loss, i.e. at least a five percent change in body weight in less than one month.

Loss of energy

You feel physically drained, sluggish, and fatigued. Your body sometimes feels heavy and performing even small tasks becomes exhausting or takes longer to complete.

Stress and anxiety

Being persistently stressed is one of the most accurate signs of depression. But how can you tell that you are depressed and not just stressed? You should look for episodes of loss of interest in life, blank stares, inability to express or feel happiness and other emotions. If you also feel empty or numb, you could be depressed.

Negative thoughts

Having depression brings negative thoughts, among them attempted suicide, as the disorder makes you despair. At this time, your only hope of ending the pain is suicide. Actually, up to 90% of all suicide victims are clinically diagnosed with depression or have had a history of drug and substance abuse. If you ever have thoughts such as, *I wish I were dead,* you are probably depressed.

Unexplained pains and aches

People often think that depression cannot result in pain, but they are wrong about this. Unexplained aches and pains are often associated with other related conditions such as constipation or diarrhea, caused by depression-linked disorders. You may experience increased physical complications such as stomach pains, aching muscles, back pains and headaches.

Chapter 3: What to Do Post Diagnosis

As soon as you have identified the problem and you know that you are going through depression, the first thing you need to do is seek help from people around you. This could be your friends, family, colleagues or anyone. It is very important that you speak out and, if the problem is really bad, you should see a doctor.

The techniques mentioned in this book are self-help and if you are seeing a doctor, the techniques should be practiced in conjunction with your doctor's advice. Basically, all the self-help tips here revolve around food for the mind, body and soul. The whole idea is to keep these three healthy by developing a good daily process. The ultimate goal of this book is to present before you the various techniques that can be easily practiced and help you draw a good daily procedure for yourself. This daily procedure, when practiced over a period of time, will become a habit even before you know it. Habits have the power to shape you and leave you in that shape for life. It is therefore very necessary that you cultivate good habits. The techniques and ideas mentioned in this book will enable you to do exactly that.

Good habits lead to great things. A glance into the lives of some of the great achievers will tell you that they all had one thing very much in common—an extremely well-disciplined life. And if you further analyze their lives, you will see how all of them had habits that took care of the three things we spoke of above—mind, body and soul. They all practiced techniques that ensured good nourishment for their mind, body and soul.

Remember, a well-nourished mind, a good body and a pure soul can never be depressed. And when you are never depressed and always looking forward to life, you will live more, give more and achieve more.

So, now, give yourself a wide smile and get ready for the next chapter, in which we will go through the 101 powerful ways to beat depression, stress, anxiety and be happy, NATURALLY!

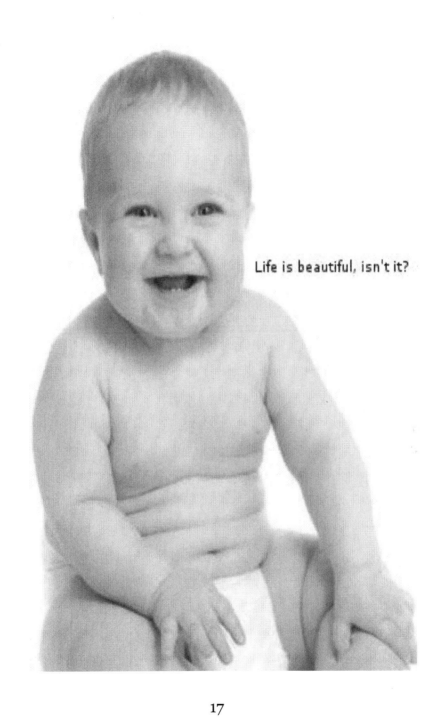

Life is beautiful, isn't it?

Chapter 4: Learn About the 101 Powerful Ways to Beat Depression, Stress, Anxiety and Be Happy Naturally.

Did you give yourself a smile? That's very good!

Someone has very rightly said that a smile is a curve that sets everything straight. So straight on we go, with that very positive thought, into the 101 powerful techniques for a healthy mind, body and soul, to free ourselves from depression, stress, anxiety and be happy forever.

1. Start your day with 2 glasses of water

Be aware that a healthy body is the foundation of a healthy mind. Start your day by activating all your internal organs and make them ready to function for the day. This can be done by drinking 2 glasses of water immediately after you wake up. Do not eat anything for at least 30 minutes once you have drunk the 2 glasses of water; just do other morning tasks within this timeline like brushing your teeth. Water will awaken your internal organs and prepare them for the day like a well-oiled machine.

Understand that it is extremely important that the internal organs are cared for and starting your day by drinking 2 glasses of water is one of the best ways of doing it.

Once you get a good start first thing in the morning, you will realize that half the battle for any upcoming challenge during the day is already won!

2. Do not skip meals during the day

Schedule your eating time to revolve around 3-4 meals per day. Regular meals help reduce chances of feeling tired or irritated, and prevent a drop in your blood sugar that also causes extreme tiredness. Skipping meals triggers persistent low blood sugar. A low sugar level in the blood also lowers the level of feel good hormones in the brain, thus episodes of depression are bound to happen.

Every meal is important but the most important of all is your breakfast. You should never skip it under any circumstances. A proper, filling breakfast can power your entire day by giving you that all-important energy boost early in the day.

3. Add some honey into your daily diet

Try adding a teaspoon of honey into your breakfast or just have it directly from the spoon. Daily intake of honey has tremendous health benefits. Besides enhancing memory power, honey also has the ability to develop and strengthen the nervous system, thus reducing stress and anxiety levels.

Ensure you buy organic and unprocessed honey only, and use as per the guidelines on the product.

4. Practice deep breathing at least once daily

Even if you can do this for just 2 minutes daily, you should. Close your eyes; breathe deeply and feel it. Place one hand on your chest and the other on your belly, and then take deep breaths through your nose and release them.

Deep breathing techniques can help you calm your mind, remove all the unwanted clutter and accumulated stress and anxiety. Try 6-10 deep and slow breaths a minute, for a duration of 10 minutes every day. But, as mentioned above, if it is difficult to take 10 minutes out, do it even if it is only for 2 minutes every day.

5. Relax every muscle whenever you get a chance

You can do this exercise at home, at your work desk on even while on the go sitting in the backseat of your car or on public transport. Close your eyes and focus on tensing and relaxing each muscle group from head to toe, for two to three seconds each. Start with the face and go down towards the neck, shoulder, chest, abdomen, thighs, calves and finally the feet. Tense each muscle group for two to three seconds and release them. One cycle should be enough each time and you can do this any number of times in a day.

This exercise will release the tension and the stress that your muscles hold, making you feel lighter and more energetic.

6. Try mindfulness – Observe nature

When was the last time you took some time out from your busy schedule to observe the beauty of nature? There are so many miracles happening all around us every second but do we have the time to stand and notice? The majority of us have lost our connection with nature.

Please do this simple task every day. For a few minutes, any time during the day, observe something like the sky, the rising sun, the moon, blooming flowers or the green trees. Do this consciously and try to absorb the impressions into you.

Being mindful helps one to keep in touch with the Creator and the vast and infinite universe energy. It is amazing how, once you get in tune with nature, nature starts flowing in you. The feeling of oneness with the universe is the ultimate bliss.

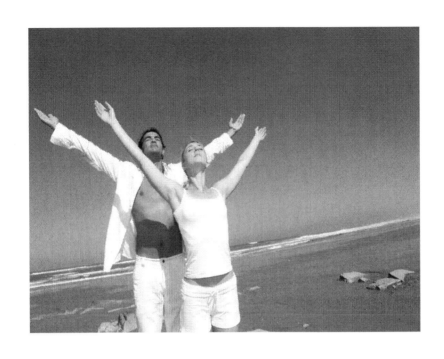

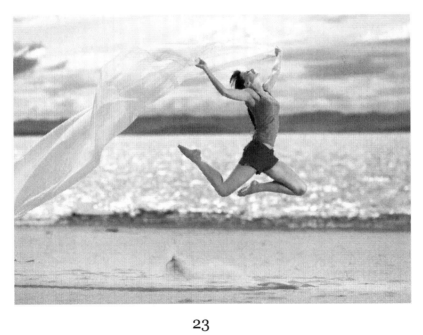

7. Exercise a bit every day

Exercises act as an active antidepressant that can increase your energy levels while minimizing fatigue. Physical activity helps trigger growth of new cells in the brain, reduces stress, and increases mood-enhancing endorphins and neurotransmitters.

Exercise for about 10-30 minutes daily to positively affect your mood. You do not need to go for heavy or strenuous exercises; even simple stretches can do wonders. The idea is to keep the body fit and flexible.

One of the easiest ways of exercising (without consciously doing it) is by shunning the lift and taking the stairs wherever possible. Also try walking instead of taking your car everywhere. If you have to take your car, try parking it at some distance from your destination so that you get to walk there and back.

8. Just before you go to sleep, do this

Some few moments before you go to sleep at night, read a few lines from a good, positive book. This will not just relax your mind but will also fill it with positivity while sleeping. Even when your body is sleeping, the mind is always awake. By feeding it with some positive words at the end of the day, you are activating it with positive energy. You will notice the effect in the morning when you wake up. You will feel light and raring to go.

In case you do not have the urge to read before you go to sleep, you can also do this - Listen to a nice song at a low volume and go to sleep (ensuring the music gets shut off automatically after some time).

Music and songs have the same effect on the mind and brain as reading positive books before going off to sleep.

9. Join a support group

We all need support in life. Even the greatest achievers in the world would not have achieved what they did if there was no support available to them in some form or other. Asking or expecting support does not mean you are weak. Neither does it mean you are dependent on someone. So never feel shy of asking for support from anyone if you need it.

There are several support groups in every city that help citizens in a variety of ways—coping with depression being one of them. Find one online and join it as you may start seeing life from a different perspective, which can be a great, positive step towards fighting depression and stress.

Have you heard about Laughter clubs? Several cities across the globe have these clubs where people assemble either daily or weekly and laugh for 10 to 15 mins. Laughter is a great medicine and a wonderful way of relieving stress and anxiety. Do check out these clubs and attend a session if you manage to find one in your city. You will not be disappointed with the outcome.

10. Help others

Try helping someone, such as a family member, your colleague at work, a stranger on the road or even someone you dislike, without expecting anything in return.

Helping others helps you get a new meaning in life and fights negative or suicidal thoughts. People do not realize how powerful it can be to do some selfless service once in a while. The smile on the face of the person receiving your help can really brighten your day and energize you to a great extent.

Help does not need to be something really big like solving someone's family problems or fixing your friend's broken relationship (it would be great if you could do that too!); it can be anything as small as offering to hold an elderly person's hand when he is climbing down stairs or lending your hand to an unknown stranger on the road who is trying to lift a heavy object. The best part about helping someone is that you really do not need to go looking for an opportunity. There are people all around us calling for help silently and in a subtle way. Just make an attempt to listen and go for it!

11. Do something new

A change in your program can make a huge difference, be it going to a museum, a rock concert, visiting an old-age home, participating in a marathon or taking a language class.

Changes can increase your level of dopamine, a brain chemical that contributes to pleasure, enjoyment, and learning.

Try to break your routine and give yourself different reasons to smile. Be on the lookout for new opportunities. These days, with so many new avenues available everywhere, finding something new to do is not very challenging. Just go on to your computer and type in 'concerts' or 'museums' or 'hobby classes' and, even before you blink your eye, you will see a list.

You should aim to do something new and different every fortnight or at least once every month. It is very important to keep gaining new insights and also give yourself new experiences every now and then.

12. Be responsible

Do not evade responsibilities even if you feel withdrawn from society. Try to get involved by doing daily chores both in the house and at work. Being responsible can act as your sense of accomplishment. Running away from responsibilities may give you a temporary relief but in the long run you will only regret it. Understand that life can only become meaningful if you live it to the fullest. And to live life to the fullest, you have to learn to undertake and fulfill all your responsibilities.

You cannot get great power unless you know how to handle it responsibly. Even if you do get power somehow and behave irresponsibly, it is only a matter of time before your power will be transferred to someone who knows how to handle it responsibly. So get responsible!

There is no greater sense of achievement than fulfilling one's own responsibilities towards someone. The immense mental peace that comes with it is a bonus.

13. Write down your experiences

Writing about one's experiences can be a great way of relieving stress. Have a journal to evaluate your daily experiences, usually after following a specific therapy or a treatment or even after making any small changes to your lifestyle. You can freely express your emotions, anger, pain or improvements in this journal. The important thing to remember here is to ensure that you just write what's in your mind and don't become obsessed about being perfect i.e. about being grammatically correct or framing the right sentences, etc. The journal is only for you and not for any publication, so just relax.

It's very important to ensure that you do not make it another stressful exercise but enjoy it and use it to de-stress.

14. Avoid caffeine, or at least reduce your intake

Taking caffeine or coffee may give your body energy but for a limited time only. It will lift your mood for a few minutes by stimulating your nervous system and that is it. Studies have shown how caffeine is responsible for a number of problems in the body including mood swings, insomnia, anxiety and depression. How wise is it to invite a long-term problem for a short-term gain?

If you cannot cut out coffee completely, at least reduce your intake. However, if you are suffering from severe depression, you should aim to keep away from caffeine and coffee completely.

15. Get Magnesium naturally

Magnesium is a good reliever of depression, and the mineral helps your body to make neurotransmitters such as serotonin.

You can get magnesium from foods such as leafy green vegetables, whole grains, nuts and legumes. Many herbs and spices such as basil, coriander, fennel seed and cumin also contain magnesium.

Avoid processed or genetically modified crops.

16. Alcohol – cut down or avoid completely

Alcohol, just like caffeine and coffee, has a stimulating effect and gives you immense pleasure and a high when you are having it. But there are long-term side effects, depression being one of them.

Social drinking once in a while may be acceptable but you should always know your limits. Your body is the best judge. Listen to it. If you are a heavy drinker, you should make every effort to cut down. For best results, consult a therapist or a counselor.

17. Highlight negative thoughts

You must have heard this many times: "Do not think negatively." However, there are times when negative thoughts just cannot be controlled. You try your level best to remain positive but your mind gets drawn towards negative thoughts. What do you do in such situations? The best way to deal with this is to welcome those thoughts and write them down. Writing down your negative thoughts can help you realize their triggers. It can also help you to identify behavioral patterns, such as those situations that lead you into negative thinking. Then you can find out ways of changing those circumstances. For instance, you may realize that interacting with specific people normally triggers your negative thinking. Once you know this, you can do something to reduce your interactions with such people.

Try this technique of highlighting your negative thoughts when you encounter this situation the next time. You will be amazed how powerful this method is.

18. Visualize

Visualization is another fabulous and powerful technique, not just for dealing with depression but also for empowering oneself with self-confidence, courage and positivity.

There are several ways of practicing visualization. One such method is explained below.

Close your eyes and picture yourself in a peaceful and serene environment that relaxes the body and soul. Take your time to imagine that these experiences are actually happening. Do the guided imagery while you focus on pleasant, positive thoughts to replace any negative images. Be in that positive zone for a few minutes. Ensure you smile when you are in that positive frame of mind with your eyes closed. Then slowly open your eyes and see how you feel. You will be relaxed and peaceful!

The thing with visualization is that your subconscious mind cannot tell the difference between you visualizing and when you are actually experiencing something great. Therefore, when visualizing the great feeling you have, your subconscious mind assumes that you are actually experiencing what you are visualizing and this is great in dealing with depression.

19. Eat superfoods

Some types of foods can directly boost your mood, such as bananas and spinach. Bananas supply your body with tryptophan, a chemical that boosts serotonin levels, as well as Vitamin B6, which improves alertness. They are a source of magnesium, which is very important in lowering anxiety. Spinach contains magnesium and folate, which improve sleeping habits and reduce agitation.

Some of the other foods that are normally referred to as superfoods are almonds, green tea, salmon, eggs, oatmeal, quinoa and lentils. These are high-nutrient foods and regular intake is great for one's health and assists in fighting depression and stress. Seaweed is another extremely nutritious food packed with natural vitamins and minerals.

20. Don't always compare yourself

One of the easiest ways of getting depressed in life is by comparing what you are and what you have with someone who has achieved more than you in life. But don't get it wrong here as sometimes it is very important to do that comparison to understand where you stand as far as your goals in life are concerned. But doing it all the time and making it a habit will depress you.

You need to understand that each one of us is special in our own way. We all have some strengths and some weaknesses. Use your strengths and work on your weaknesses. Figure out where you are in life and where you have to go. Compare yourself to yourself.

You should also never compare and judge others. Everyone is fighting some unknown battle we just don't know about. Thus the parameters by which you compare will never be the same.

21. Use Positive Affirmations

Have you ever noticed how your mood lightens up when someone appreciates you? Imagine receiving that appreciation every 15 minutes of your life. Yes, it is possible! Just surround yourself with positive affirmations; basically feel good quotes telling you how wonderful you are.

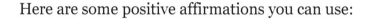

Here are some positive affirmations you can use:

"I am the best."

"I handle every situation confidently."

"I see the best in everyone."

"I am the luckiest person on this planet."

"I am always in the right place at the right time."

Make these affirmations your screen saver. Make a photo frame and keep it in your bedroom so that the first thing you see in the morning is a positive affirmation. Keep it in your car or on your work desk in your office and see how it benefits you.

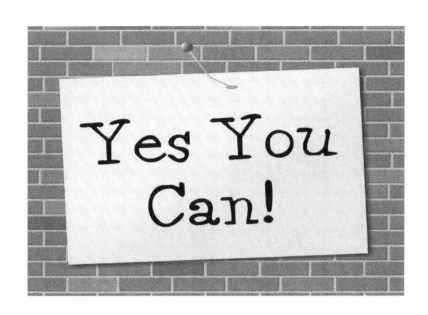

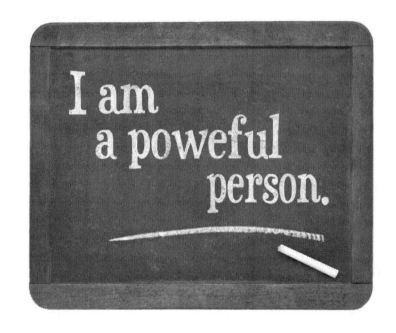

22. Do the right thing

However tough it may be, always do the right thing. Doing right will help you boost or strengthen your self-esteem. Conversely, trying to take the easy way out by doing a wrong thing will harm you in the long run and severely affect your self-esteem. Remember, it is better not to do anything than to do a wrong thing in life.

Also avoid being judgmental and concentrate on you. Make the right choices that will benefit you in the long run. Do not look for short-term gains but always aim for long-term strategies and be in the right game!

23. Avoid negative people

Demotivating people can actually ruin your mood or frustrate your efforts in fighting stress or depression.

We all have friends or relatives who always complain about everything in life. Keep away from them. If you take a glance into the lives of such negative people, you will see a whole web of problems in their lives. And if you analyze their issues, you will realize that the majority of their problems are their own doing. A little bit of positive thinking will solve a lot of their problems. Limit the time you spend with such people.

Unsupportive people, mean people, and negative thinkers will only make your depression worse. Likewise, avoid websites, magazines, TV programs, or radio shows that promote negative thinking.

24. Learn to pause at times

Life these days, for most of us, has become extremely hectic. We are all trying to do several things at the same time. Many people get into depression just trying to keep pace with the life around them. So what is the solution? Well, learn to pause a bit at times when you feel the pace is too much. For instance, you have just come into the office and your colleague tells you about a client issue that needs to be sorted immediately. Before you log into your system to get on to the issue, just pause. Take a deep breath and give yourself some time for the news to sink in. Once it does, get on to the issue with full vigor and complete focus.

Practice this technique and see how you are able to handle issues with much better mental clarity. Extend this technique to pausing in other areas of your life as well.

25. Respect relationships

We all want people around us, especially our close family members, to respect us. Gaining respect is very important to boosting our self-esteem and confidence. However, as they say, "You can only get respect if you give respect." Hence you should treat everyone in the same way you want everyone to treat you. Respect your parents, your siblings, your relatives, your girlfriend, spouse and your children.

Your family can play a very important role in ensuring your happiness and keeping you away from depression, but you need to ensure that the bond is kept strong for them to help you and be there for you always. Mutual respect is one of the key ingredients in ensuring a strong, life-long relationship with anyone.

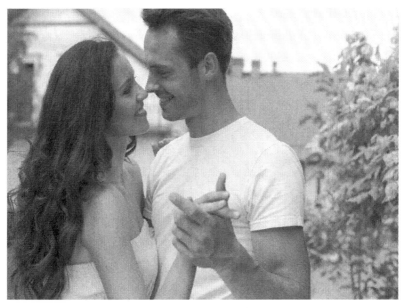

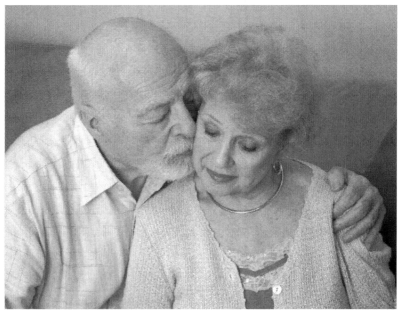

26. Get 6-8 hours of sleep

Good sleep for a minimum of 6 to 8 hours is a must for the body to re-energize. You must have learnt that lack of sleep can cause depression. Try to adopt a regular sleeping schedule whereby you sleep at the same time and wake up at the same time ensuring you sleep for 6-8 hours.

It is not difficult to get into this routine. Just a little bit of discipline is required.

27. Interact with people

When you are depressed, you have a tendency to want to stay alone. Kindly abstain from this because it only makes things worse. It is best to interact with friends, play with your kids, or just spend time with people doing fun things. The more time you spend alone, the worse the depression will be.

Interacting with long-lost friends by finding out where they are and calling them up is a great way of re-energizing yourself. Try this today—make a list of all your school and college friends. Then reach out to people who are in touch with you and ask them for contact numbers of the ones you have lost touch with. Surprise your long-lost friends by calling them up. You will be amazed how happy they will be to hear from you. The re-connection after years can sometimes work like magic for your spirits. Whenever you are down and need to lift yourself up, use this technique. Speaking to an old friend and sharing a laugh is the best way to get back into the rhythm of life.

28. Don't try being perfect every time

Perfection is good but obsession with perfection can kill you. Trying to be perfect every time may paralyze and hinder you from meeting the standard as you tend to be anxious every time.

Being carried away with perfectionism will not just hurt you but also other people connected to your life. Be dedicated to doing your best in whatever you do but do not be obsessed with being perfect. You must know that nothing in life is perfect and as human beings, we all have our imperfections. As hard as this may be to accept, the earlier you accept it the better it is for you. As a general rule, when you do something, just aim to finish it in the best possible way. You can always go back and improve it. By doing this, you are not putting that pressure on you to be perfect every time.

29. Eat Omega-3 Fatty Acids

Based on research, depression can be triggered by insufficient intake of omega-3 fatty acids too.

Try to include fish, which is high in EPA and DHA omega-3 fatty acids, in your diet. Eat fish such as sardines, sturgeon, tuna, lake trout, bluefish, herring, mackerel, anchovies and salmon.

If possible, you should try eating wild-caught salmon 2-3 times a week.

30. Incorporate scents

This concept is referred to as aromatherapy, and has shown to sooth depression symptoms. You must surely have noticed how a good smell elevates mood.

Surrounding yourself with specific scents like vanilla, which is quite grounding, can provide you the comfort you need. There are several ways in which you can use scents—room spray, massage, bath etc.

31. Warm up

Depression is easily fought through relaxation. The best way to warm up is by soaking yourself in the steam of hot shower, taking a bubble bath, or taking other relaxing baths that you prefer.

You can enjoy a hot cup of tea or cocoa at bath time if desired.

32. Increase Folate intake naturally

Lack of folate in your diet or low levels of vitamin B can worsen depression. Folate deficiency also leads to several other problems.

Ensure your diet has enough foods containing folate, which occurs naturally in a wide variety of foods such as green leafy vegetables, fruits, beans, dairy and poultry products and seafood.

33. Make a list and combat

Stress and anxiety are caused by various reasons and often we are aware of them but just don't have a plan to address the factors. So here is what you need to do. Pick up a pen and a paper and sit down. Now think of all the reasons that are the causes of stress in your life. Once you have the list ready, write down the least you can do to address these factors. Keep adding to that list every day and within a week you will have a plan ready to act on. Check each one of them as you handle them. The more items you tick off the list the higher the chances that you will start feeling better about yourself.

This is a wonderful technique that will surely give you results if you follow it thoroughly and take action accordingly.

34. Do what you enjoy, regularly

Do motivating stuff such as listening to music, writing or chatting with a friend as you carry out various activities.

Come up with a list of things that you enjoy doing that can be done within the time you have available. The more you have fun and enjoy life the less you will be depressed. Even when you don't feel like doing anything enjoyable, just force yourself to do it because, after some time, you will find yourself having fun. Even if you just smile once that is good enough and is a step in the right direction.

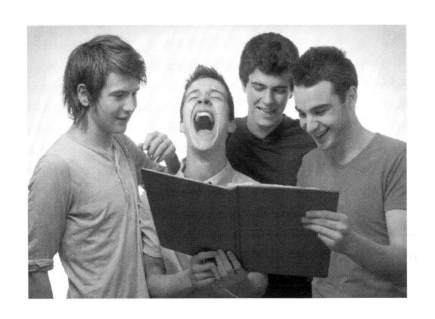

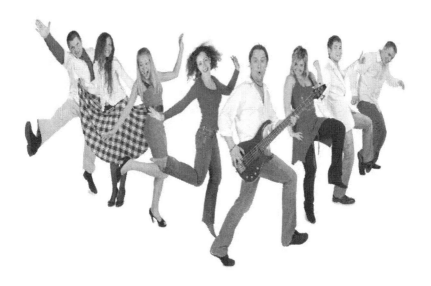

35. Get enough Vitamin B6 through natural foods

You need vitamin B6 so as to produce neurotransmitters such as dopamine and serotonin. The vitamin supports nervous system, proper maintenance of red blood cells and improvement of the immune system.

Eat plenty of pistachio nuts, sunflower seeds, tuna, and dried fruit such as prunes, bananas and avocados.

36. Don't be over ambitious

The higher your expectations the higher the likelihood you will be depressed if things don't work as expected. This type of self-imposed stress is brought about by your unrealistic attitude towards issues. Keep your expectations within manageable levels if you don't want disappointments that could probably make you depressed. It is natural to feel that everything will work in your favor but you must be realistic too, and not try to be overambitious about your projects.

37. Try counselling

If your condition keeps on relapsing, it is not a bad idea to obtain help from a qualified expert. Visit your health provider and explain your depression symptoms, among them any bad feelings or negative thoughts. Sometimes even a general talk with someone who has come out of depression can be invaluable. You should never be shy of seeking help and counseling. Just speak out!

38. Handle failures positively

Failures are the stepping stones to success—you must have heard this so many times. To stumble and fall is human nature, so find a way of moving on. Be your own best friend, and find ways in which your friends or parents may support you in your failures. Only focus on the optimism and opportunities that can come from your experiences.

Once you learn from failures and see them as opportunities, you will be pleasantly surprised at the various opportunities at your disposal. Failure can, at times, teach you a lot more than success. You will realize this, years later when you look back. It is therefore very important to learn to handle failures positively, see the bigger picture and not get depressed in any way.

39. Ensure you have chromium in your diet

Chromium is extremely useful in fighting 'atypical' depression. Symptoms for this type of depression include weight gain, fatigue, sleepiness, and carb cravings.

Adequate intake of chromium through foods like broccoli, whole grain bread, bananas, and mushrooms is recommended.

40. Do moderate activities

Try to do physical activities that are of moderate intensity to avoid overworking yourself. Moderate exercises can bring more mental benefits without much sweating.

Another approach is to choose exercises that are rhythmic and continuous such as stationary biking, swimming, dancing and walking.

41. Adopt healthier motivation habits

To encourage yourself and boost your self-worth, highlight benefits you stand to get from changing your perception or achieving a set goal. Save this list in a place where you can refer to it daily, such as on a fridge or at a workplace.

Also, try to concentrate on your hobbies, which actually boost your mood automatically. Subscribe to daily motivational quotes to inspire yourself. Reading motivational quotes can be a very powerful exercise, not just for the conscious but even for the subconscious mind.

42. Take a self-appreciation break

Reserve some time, say 2 to 5 minutes daily, when you just relax, slowly take a deep breath, and then focus on three things you can actually appreciate about yourself.

This may include the way you can inspire people through music or poetry or how you can make others happy through your talent in comedy. We all have some hidden talents in us. Identify what it is in you, bring it out and showcase it to the world.

43. Change your look once in a while

Change the way you look once in a while by sporting a moustache or a goatee if you are a male. If you are a female, try a different hairstyle. See how people notice the difference and enjoy the attention.

Always dress nicely, as looking good can actually attract people. Also, when you are well dressed, you tend to be more confident. Observe good hygiene and adopt a nice walking posture. Try to maintain eye contact, standing up straight or keeping your head up, to boost confidence.

44. Make your dinner time a celebration every day

There is no better place in the world to get de-stressed than a dining table with food and family. Make your dinner a special occasion daily. Switch off all technology—i.e. television, mobile phones, and internet—during dinner. Light a candle in the middle to give the feeling of celebration. You should do this every day. This will not just bring the family closer but will also provide a platform every day for everyone to speak out and express their thoughts.

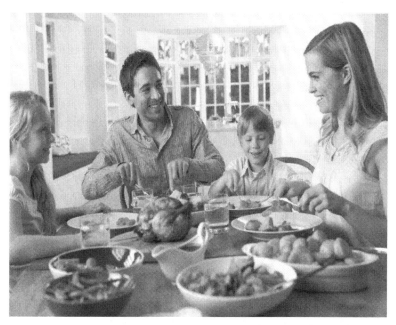

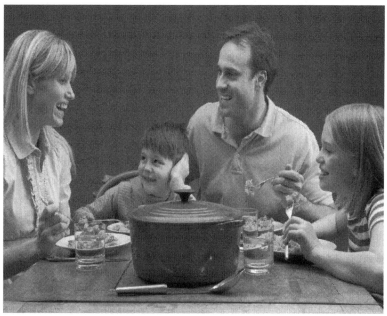

45. Be informed

Learn more about depression to avoid getting back into similar experiences. You should motivate your family to be conversant with the condition to help them understand you while they offer support. The more you understand the symptoms and techniques to keep away from depression, the better you will be in actually keeping it away from you.

Hopefully, this book will help you achieve this as our purpose here is exactly that—to get the information across to you and to make you aware of the various techniques to help you.

Be informed so that you can help not only yourself but also anyone around who is showing signs and symptoms of depression and stress. Your proactive approach may help prevent a life from going astray and bring it back to normal.

46. Prioritize tasks

Our lives are so hectic these days that we have to multi-task. Multi-tasking is one of the prime reasons for stress.

When you have a number of things to do, make a list and assign priority to the tasks. Though every task may seem urgent, in reality, if you analyze and look into the consequences of not doing a certain task, you will see that only a few are actually really urgent and need to be completed first. The others can wait.

So prioritize and do the most important task first and the others later. This will help you reduce stress levels as the pressure of multi-tasking will come down dramatically.

47. Live in the moment

The past is over; the future is not yet here. What you have is the present. Live it.

Thinking about incidences in the past will not change them. It will only spoil your present. Yes, sometimes it is difficult to let go of the past but you have to make an effort. Please understand that you can only create something new in the present, nothing in the past. Similarly, worrying about the future continuously is also futile. Concentrate on doing your best in the present moment and your future will automatically shape up.

Practice living in the present and enjoy what life has to offer you in the current moment.

48. Think positively, always

No matter what the situation is, however hard the circumstances are, always, always, always think positively. So much has been said about positive thinking everywhere that we don't think we need to stress it more here.

People who think positively, attract positivity and, hence, lead good lives. Concentrate on positive thoughts and see the way your life changes.

49. Keep your options open in life

Don't be rigid in your thoughts. Be open to change and enjoy what life has to offer. As you grow and mature, you will realize that the options to reach your goals are varied. You may plan something for months and suddenly you may see a different and an easier way. What will you do? You will come across several such crossroads in life where you will need to choose whether to stick to your ways or try something different that is on offer. Be open and have the courage to explore, of course after calculating all the risks.

Under no circumstances should you get into something that will take away your mental peace and frustrate you. So keep your options open but explore wisely.

50. Schedule tasks

Another great technique for managing your work-related stress is by scheduling tasks.

Structure your time for each task and use sticky notes to serve as reminders. You can also use other planners like email calendars or alarms to stay organized.

Staying organized is extremely important to ensure you are not putting too much pressure on yourself at any point in time and, thus, not stressing yourself.

51. Take personal care

It is very important to take time out daily for your personal needs. Do not ignore yourself for work. Remember, you are working for a living, not living for working.

If you are on a treatment plan, take time out and stick to it, ensuring that you attend all appointments and sessions.

52. Get diagnosed early – do not wait

Just like any other health issue, getting diagnosed early in case of depression can help tremendously in its treatment. Please do not ignore the signs. Avoid waiting for too long before getting diagnosed or treated, as doing this worsens the condition.

53. Laugh

A quick way to lighten your load and melt stress and anxiety is to either smile or laugh out loud. A number of studies have revealed that when you let out a giggle, the level of stress hormones goes down.

Laughter also helps boost your immunity and lowers blood pressure and cholesterol levels. Most doctors will tell you, "Laughter is the best medicine," and it is 100% true.

54. De-clutter the brain

Be aware that physical clutter contributes to mental clutter, i.e. a messy workplace can hinder effective relaxation and make work appear never-ending. Reserve 5 minutes to tidy up your work area or living space, as doing this helps you think rationally.

Always keep your workplace, home and surroundings clean.

55. Express gratitude

It is very important in life to express gratitude for all the good things around you and to all the good people around you. Never miss an opportunity to say, "Thank you," to someone. Also express your gratitude to the wonderful nature around you, the sun for coming out every day, the trees moving in the fresh breeze, the flowers for bringing color and fragrance into your life.

Research has shown that, when stressed, expressing gratitude can actually work. But you don't need to wait until you are stressed to express gratitude. Just get into the habit of appreciating life and all the wonderful things around you.

56. Eat whole-grain carbs

Complex carb helps monitor the level of serotonin, or the feel good hormone that helps the mind to remain calm. Eat whole carbs like oats, cassava and brown rice to counteract occasional cravings. These foods also contain fiber, which slows down digestion and makes you feel fuller and relaxed.

Avoid consuming simple sugars and refined foods such as baked food, sweet snacks, French fries and other comfort foods.

57. Meditate

Meditating helps boost the amount of grey matter in your brain and, thus, helps lower stress levels. When you meditate, you're able to understand how your mind triggers depression-provoking thoughts. To fight negative thoughts, you need to understand the brain's thought patterns.

Research has shown that meditation can also help improve brain power and intelligence, empowering you with more tools to help you go through life smoothly, keeping away from depression and stress.

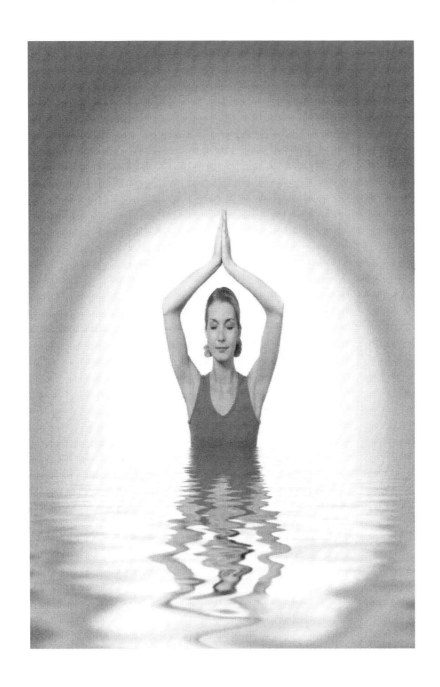

58. Make a vision board

If thinking of the future appears intimidating, create a vision board that depicts the fun side of your possibilities or projects to come. You can make your own or use an e-vision board using Pinterest.

Ensure you put the vision board somewhere you can see easily it in the morning to remind you that your future is not as bleak as you think and to evoke positive feelings.

59. Play around

Sometimes you need to view life as a small kid or as an animal. Play to relieve your stress. Learn to play even when business commitments and deadlines consume your time. Try taking your dog out or babysit to clear anxiety from the mind. Playing with kids can be a great stress reliever. When you are with children, just become like one of them and enjoy the fun.

60. Set a quiet time

Schedule a few minutes every day when you should fully disconnect, with your cell phone off and away from TV and internet too. Research has shown that stress and anxiety can be worsened by noise and bright lights from TV, phones and other equipment. You need some silent time among all the difficulties that may be going on in your life.

Each time you have a quiet period, you rejuvenate and get some peace of mind that gives you the strength to deal with anything you may be going through.

61. Have a worry period

We all have worries in life and that's the hard fact. Running away is not the solution. Facing it will solve it. But worrying all the time will complicate it.

Try this technique. Allocate a few minutes to consider your worries and miseries. Within this worry period, think about all possible scenarios or outcomes, create a game plan and figure out your next course of action. To avoid being carried away in thought, ensure you allocate a specific amount of time like 15 minutes, after which you will get back to doing your daily activities. During the day, if you have any worries just put them aside and think about them during that 15-minute worry period. This will ensure that you do not make your depression worse by worrying all the time, as it will reduce the amount of time you worry drastically.

62. Take a break from the routine

This is perhaps one of the most important techniques to de-stress—take a break from the routine. There are times when you are not feeling great and need to make important decisions. If possible, take a break and postpone making any decisions until you feel better.

You can never make a good decision if you are not in the right frame of mind. So break away, if possible, and come back. This break can be for 5 mins, 5 hours, 5 days, 5 weeks or even more depending upon the situation.

63. Hang out

Social support can help you de-stress as it stimulates synthesis of the hormone oxytocin, which fights stress and anxiety.

Make some time for friends, to obtain vital support when the going gets tougher. Go for a walk, go to the movies or have a talk at a coffee shop with someone you admire.

64. Knit

Research has shown that knitting can help boost mood, induce relaxation and make you forget pain you may be feeling. Fight stress by doing a repetitive, bilateral and rhythmic activity, which functions in a similar manner as meditation.

65. Go gardening

Gardening is another great way of getting close to nature. And the more you are close to nature the better your ability to embrace life and stay positive becomes. Nature has that amazing, life-enhancing energy.

Try to do some gardening work whenever you get a chance. Research has shown that the process of planting and growing can help relieve stress and anxiety.

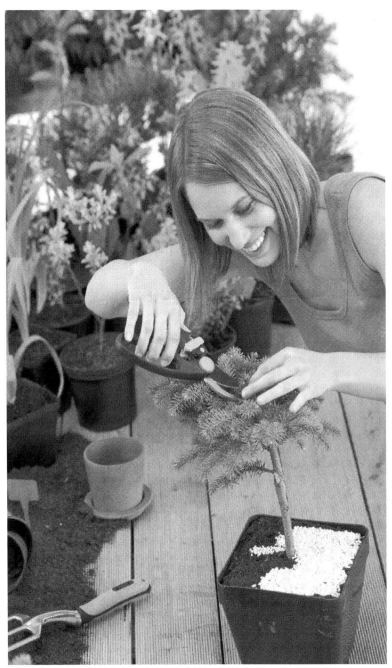

66. Use Internet Social Networks sparingly and wisely

Social media has great benefits but, if used heavily and insensibly, it can create problems too. Many people use social media to promote a non-existent self-image, which can unconsciously make them compare themselves to others. This can trigger self-loathing, insecurity, feelings of superiority or being misplaced.

Hence, be aware of your limits and spend time online wisely. Do not try to be someone you are not and be honest on your public profiles and posts.

67. Live your life and not someone else's

Stress and depression are also triggered by the desire to please others, say your parents, co-workers, friends, spouse, or children. You should stop this self-destruction by setting boundaries when it comes to negative influences in your life while trying to please others.

Follow your own dreams and aspirations despite what people think of you. However, you should also be realistic and only take calculated risks. For example, you have a good job and you think of becoming an entrepreneur. You cannot just quit overnight and set up a shop. You should research the market you want to be in, get up-to-date information, speak to people in that area, understand the profit margin and rate of returns, arrange for investments, set up bank accounts—and only when you are ready with a complete plan and a back-up plan, should you think about quitting your job and moving ahead.

So go for your dreams and live your life but do not be reckless. Behave sensibly.

68. Plan ahead

Plan your activities and thoughts using a to-do list, to reduce stress while boosting productivity. This is not just for the bigger things in life but also for every little thing that you do daily. For instance, make lunch ahead of time, pack a gym bag and leave it by the door, lay out clothes the previous night deciding what to wear the next day, so you save time in the morning.

Planning helps in giving you peace of mind because you know everything is in order.

69. Pick a Goal

There are two types of goals: short-term and long-term.

Try to set up both in your life but ensure you don't become too obsessed with long-term goals. Try to sync your short-term goals with the long-term ones so that you don't really have to think about the long-term goals. Just work away on the short-term goals and, before you know it, your long-term goals will be achieved. For example, your long-term goal is to clear your final exams with 90% marks. Keep your short terms goals as, "Study 2 chapters every day without fail." (Just an example.) If you diligently follow your short-term goals and meet them daily, there is no way your long-term goal will not be achieved.

It's important to note that there is no need for your short-terms goals to have any long-term vision. For instance, your short-term goal is to play football for 45 minutes every day. You do not need to attach any long-term goal to it. But if you have long-term goals, it is recommended that you break them into short-term ones as it becomes easier to work on them and achieve them.

Achievement of a goal is a huge morale booster. It can help fight depression and stress in a huge way.

70. Study spirituality and science

Even if you're a diehard atheist or agnostic, books on astronomy, astrology or spirituality can help you realize the big, cosmic, universal picture. You're bound to regain your sense of comfort and mastery in your life. Once you come to terms with the enormity of your world, you will take life less seriously.

Also pick up books on science and study the back-end occurrences and events of things that were always a mystery to you (for instance, the evolution of the universe).

Sometimes, trying to correlate science and spiritually can really enlighten you to the wider scheme of things in the divine order. The more you know about the vastness of the cosmos, the less you will feel worried about yourself.

71. Find happiness everywhere – make an effort

Realize that happiness takes effort, practice and vigilance, thus you should take a hard look at life. Aim to be peaceful by taking things slowly, as you have all time in the world. Eliminate negative people, change your ambitions and modify your behavior for the better.

Find happiness and happiness will find you!

72. Swim

Swimming helps shrink the panic and grief as it combines different techniques such as repetitiveness, breathing, and stroke mechanics. Research has shown that people who engage in three sessions of rigorous anaerobic exercises are able to treat depression just as well as those who take medicine.

73. Record your fun

This should not be a very difficult thing to do these days with cameras on every phone. Take pictures, clips and make a movie. Capture the good times!

Recording your fun moments and referring to them at times of stress and heavy workload is a great way of de-stressing yourself. If possible, you should make a physical album of the pictures. You should go back to your albums once in a while as this will let you enjoy your moments of delight once again. These happy moments are what counts when you are depressed and sad.

74. Count accomplishments

This is one thing that most of us never do. We achieve so many things in our lives everyday but we never give credit to ourselves for them because we feel they are too small to count. For instance, you reached the office 5 minutes early today. Isn't that an accomplishment? Of course it is. Count all such small and large accomplishments you made during the day before you go to bed. It will help you build strength and confidence for the next day.

75. Drink a power smoothie

For your breakfast, blend a smoothie made from strawberries, pineapples, collard greens, kale, chard or spinach. Then add in a probiotic, a powdery mix that contains healthy bacteria to boost digestion and enhance intestinal heath.

Your intestines have 500 million neurons, and a healthy gut is as important as the brain.

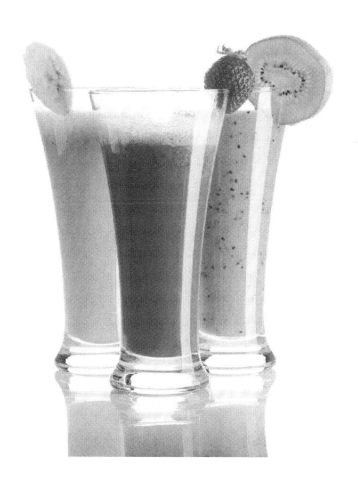

76. Avoid gluten

Gluten in wheat and grains is responsible for inflammation, a condition that affects the body alongside the brain. These foods affect brain cells and alter your mood, leading to anxiety, depression and other disorders.

Eggs, fish, fruits, vegetables and grains like quinoa, rice, millet, and corn are examples of gluten-free foods.

77. Get Sun-shine regularly

Sun is the reason why we are all alive today. The energy from the sun helps plants create food for themselves and, in the process, they take in carbon dioxide and release oxygen into the atmosphere, thus maintaining life on this planet.

Research has shown that sunshine is vital for every living organism. A regular dosage of sunshine helps fight stress and depression. Sunbathing once in a while is also a great way of rejuvenating one's mind and body.

78. Pray

Praying can be powerful if you do it with full devotion and faith. Even if you are not religious, you can pray and direct your prayers to the universal consciousness. Include someone else in your prayers, too, at times. You don't need to spend a lot of time praying. Even a 2-minute prayer done with complete honesty can do miracles for your soul.

79. Get distracted

Find ways of escaping the tempting or anxious thoughts by taking a walk, having a cup of hot tea or taking a refreshing bath. Put the work or stressing tasks away and take a nap for 15-20 minutes, or attempt a crossword puzzle. Once you have calmed down, you can return to the suspended tasks.

Just as sometimes you have to 'break yourself' to 'make yourself', similarly, at times, you have to 'get distracted' to 'get connected'.

80. Understand your condition – be honest

Understanding the symptoms and understanding your condition can be two different things. You may be aware of all the symptoms and might be going through some too, but somehow you do not want to acknowledge it. Please be honest and face the reality always. It is far easier to solve a problem when you understand and acknowledge the gravity of it.

Once you understand your condition and take measures to come out of it, assess your progress honestly at regular intervals. If you are not getting the desired relief, speak out and adopt new ways.

81. Drink Green Tea

This herbal tea, which is now easily available in every store across the globe, contains a variety of enzymes, which work to boost your mood.

Green tea lowers stress levels as well as improving the levels of other neurotransmitters such as dopamine.

Add a green tea bag to a cup of hot water and drink it daily.

82. Try Holy Basil

Holy basil is a plant used extensively in India. This herb is effective in reducing stress by hindering the build-up of cortisol. It can also improve cerebral circulation and memory, while at the same time relieving cloudy thinking and general mental fog.

A couple of holy basil leaves can be used in cooking. If you are suffering from severe depression and are taking medication, please consult your doctor before doing this. Also, if you are trying to get pregnant, already pregnant or about to have surgery, you should avoid holy basil.

83. Treat insomnia with Valerian

If you are suffering from insomnia or sleep disorders (both of which are a cause and a symptom of depression) and have been using traditional sleeping pills, check with your doctor if you can switch to Valerian herb.

Valerian dried root (which is the most natural form) can be consumed by dissolving one teaspoon in a glass of hot water to relieve insomnia. However, you should check with your doctor or health advisor before you intake Valerian as you do not want the herbs to clash with any existing medicines or medical condition.

84. Be financially smart

A lot of people get into depression due to money worries, not being financially sound. It is actually not very difficult to be financially smart and make smart savings and investments. You really don't need to cut down on anything. Just research a bit before you spend your dollar. For instance, if you want to get a mortgage, check the website of every available bank for their interest rate and service charges. Do not go by the advice of anyone and select a bank blindly. Calculate the EMI of every bank, taking into account their special offers, if any. Then approach the top 3 banks offering the best rate and cut your deal with the one that is offering the best of all. A good deal on a mortgage can save you hundreds of dollars every year!

Similarly, for your daily shopping, find out which store offers the best deals. Most people do not want to go to the trouble of researching and end up spending more. Remember, a dollar saved is like a dollar earned.

Also take advantage of every loyalty card in the market. These days, many of them have phone apps so you do not even need to carry the cards in your wallet.

85. Get active in life

Your work will fill up most parts of your day and your life. If it is boring and mundane, try making it interesting and active. For instance, if you are a customer service agent, you will be taking calls throughout the day, speaking to clients. This can not only be stressful but can also become a boring, repetitive task. Introduce something new into it like a novel way of greeting and signing off. Instead of just, "Good morning," try saying this, with a wide smile on your face, "Good morning. Hope you are having a wonderful morning and looking forward to a blissful day! What can I do for you?" or "Good morning, what can I do to make this day eventful for you? I am at your service." Most clients (even if they are angry about something for which they have phoned you) will tone down and speak to you in a friendly way if you introduce yourself in a 'not so normal' manner.

Apart from work, try to fill your breaks and after work time with activities that you enjoy—namely cycling, dancing, sports, working out at the gym.

86. Realize how others affect you

Your family, friends or coworkers can change your mental state and probably worsen or relax your current state of mind. Find out those people who trigger anxiousness, doubts, and fears; and those who help you gain perspective. Understanding this will help you in dealing with such people.

You should also know that, just as others affect you, you affect others. Be kind and understanding in your dealings with people so that you don't become a reason for depression and stress in someone else.

87. Practice Yoga

Yoga has gained tremendous acceptability across the globe over the years due to the immense benefits associated with it, so much so that the United Nations decided to celebrate Yoga by declaring the summer solstice (longest day of the year) every year as the 'International Day of Yoga'.

Daily practice of Yoga balances the mind and body. One can reap tremendous health benefits from it, including better resistance to diseases, clarity of mind, improved memory and healthier nervous system.

If you are beginner, you should join a Yoga class and learn from an expert instructor. It is very important that the Yoga postures and techniques are done the right way to get the maximum benefits.

88. Run

Running relaxes and boosts your overall body and mind performance since it triggers production of endorphins, the chemicals that fight anxiety.

To get started, begin with 15-30 minutes of jogging every day and progress from there. Running is the easiest form of physical activity that you can engage in to fight depression and stress.

89. Love yourself

Love the way you are. You may not be perfect but no one in this world is. Give yourself a pat on the back once in a while for your achievements in life. When you start loving yourself, you will realize the importance of being happy. And when you find reasons to be happy, life will begin to flow within you.

Love is a powerful tool that can conquer anything. Bring an abundance of love into your life and see how depression, stress and anxiety will never touch you!

90. Polish your intelligence

To stay ahead in the game, especially in your workplace, in order to ensure no missed deadlines or late evenings and stressful meetings, you need to be a bit smarter and more intelligent than others. The good news is you don't need to be born intelligent; you can always improve your intelligence.

Reading is a great way to exercise the brain. Pick up books on your chosen subject and gain as much knowledge as you can. Another way of improving your intelligence is by solving puzzles and playing crosswords. You should do these things regularly so that you give your brain enough exercise and stimulate it, thus keeping it away from stress as well.

Please check our book titled – Brain: 51 Powerful Ways to Improve Brain Power, Enhance Memory, Intelligence and Concentration NATURALLY!

This book is available world-wide – see details on the last page of this book.

91. Eat almonds

These nuts are rich in zinc, a mineral that helps balance mood. Almonds also contain healthy fats and iron, a nutrient that inhibits brain fatigue.

Besides helping fight depression, almonds offer a variety of other health benefits, being a nutritionally rich food.

92. Switch to herbal teas

If you are currently on medication for depression, check with your doctor if you can switch to the different varieties of herbal teas for enhancing your mood naturally.

There are various options available in the market—St John's Wort, which can be consumed in the form of tea, can be a good stress reliever. Ginseng tea is great for lifting your mood as well. Catnip herb tea is good for calming your nerves, improving digestion and aiding good sleep.

Please note you should not try any of these without checking with your doctor as, although these are good, natural ways to relieve stress and depression, your doctor is the right person to tell you if you should really go for them depending upon your condition.

93. Eat more blueberries

Many people ignore these blue fruits probably due to their color. The fruit contains phytonutrients, vitamins, and useful antioxidants, all of which all combat anxiety and depression symptoms.

So the next time you do your weekly grocery shopping, ensure blueberries are on your list of things to buy.

94. Learn to forgive and move on

No matter how good you are to everyone you meet, you will always come across people who will hurt you—sometimes intentionally and sometimes unintentionally.

Learn to forgive. Holding on to the hurt will only harm you. Once you forgive and move on, all the toxic energy is released, which will eventually make you feel lighter.

Forgiveness is the sign of the brave. A weak person cannot forgive but can only think about revenge.

Try this next time you are hurt by someone. Just close your eyes and say, "I forgive you." You will experience a genuine feeling of peace and calmness.

If you are carrying ill feelings for someone in your heart for something that they did to you years ago, the time to forgive is now. Throw that baggage out of your heart and off your shoulders for life.

Forgiveness for others can go a long way in helping you lead a stress-free life. Just try it!

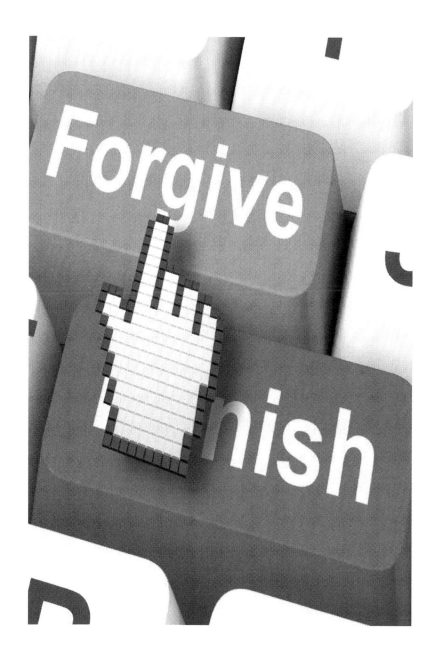

95. Stop smoking

You are really lucky if you are a non-smoker. Cigarette smoke contains a harmful product referred to as nicotine. Despite being a stimulant, nicotine increases levels of anxiety and depression.

If you are a heavy smoker, first try cutting down the number of cigarettes you smoke. If you find it difficult and the craving is too severe, get support. There are several support groups and you can easily find one by doing a brief Google search on the internet.

By quitting cigarettes, you are not just moving away from the problems of depression and stress but also from all the other dangerous illnesses, as smoking affects every part of the body.

96. Improve quality of sleep

It is not just important to have 6 to 8 hours of sleep but also very important to have good quality of sleep.

If you normally have problems sleeping, try to relax 30 minutes before going to bed. Try techniques such as taking several breaths, listening to your favorite music or taking a relaxing bath. You can also undertake mental exercise like playing Scrabble, crossword puzzles or other stress-free exercises.

When you sleep, ensure there is no light falling on your eyes. Light exposure results in suppression of melatonin production, which controls our sleep-wake times. Thus, for a healthy, good night's sleep, ensure the room is dark.

97. Accept uncertainty as part of life

You must understand that life will have its ups and downs. Be ready for it. Respond to situations rather than react. Understand the difference between responding and reacting. Reaction is always a sudden outburst without applying logic but response is a mature answer to a situation. Responding to a situation will help in controlling the damage.

Thus dreadful events cannot be avoided but they can be controlled if you act in a mature way. Realize that being worried will not hinder the occurrence of dangerous events.

98. Postpone worries

If stress and worries attack you during times of study, a working period, or other social activity, just close your eyes and take your thoughts to some wonderful memory—this could be an achievement at school, recognition at work or a fun event at a family occasion. Basically, take your thoughts away to a nice feeling for some time. When you open your eyes, you will feel a bit more relaxed. Concentrate on the present and tell yourself, "I will not worry about the situation now. Let me postpone it."

This technique of postponing your worries will ensure that you do not remain worried all the time about something. Please understand that no situation will become better by itself simply by worrying about it all the time.

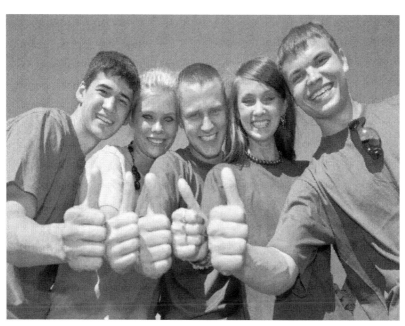

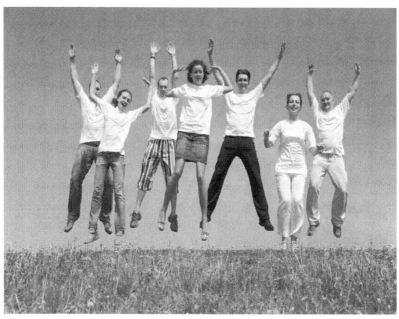

99. Explore safe remedies

Try this technique if you feel there are too many worries in your life. Classify your worries into solvable and unsolvable ones, based on how real or dangerous they are. If you think all your worries are equal in nature, take assistance from someone close to help you classify them. Never feel too shy to ask for support. Once you've classified your concerns, consider the likelihood of the feared events occurring and possible solutions in case of their occurrence. This classification and further analysis will help you deal with worries in a much better way.

One more thing—learn to accept your emotions so that anxiety episodes don't overwhelm you. Explore your options and safe remedies.

100. Welcome the worst

A person who is always willing and ready to welcome the worst can never, ever get into any kind of depression or stress, simply because he is prepared both mentally and physically to deal with life and its many challenges. Life will never overwhelm such an individual.

Learn to see the larger scheme of things in life. There is always a bigger design somewhere and the incidents in our lives are only minor dots that will connect at some point in the future. Wait for that moment for the dots to connect instead of worrying and getting depressed about the situation now.

Look back at some of the challenges in your life. In most cases you will notice that your worst fears never came true. And that is how it will always be. But be prepared and welcome the worst. You might actually be surprised that it is not as bad as you had thought!

And Lastly

101. Prepare for Monday

Get ready for Monday. For most people, Mondays tend to be stressful due to piled up tasks from the previous week, and it may be a big challenge to jump right back in.

To fight Monday anxiety, reduce your tasks by Friday afternoon to as few as possible. Keep Mondays light and, wherever possible, try not to schedule important meetings on that day. Plan your day in such a way that you are able to leave on time.

Well, you should plan all your days in such a way, but do make a special effort for Mondays.

Chapter V: All about Clinical Depression

In the last chapter, we talked about the diagnosis and 101 ways to treat depression. In this chapter, we would like to discuss other forms of depression which are more severe or acute, in other words, 'clinical depression.'

What is clinical depression?

Depression is a state of mind which can range from temporary and mild episodes of sadness to acute and persistent types which are called clinical depression. They can also be termed as a major depressive disorder. This kind of depression is not similar to the ones caused by situations such as the death of a close relative or any medical condition like hyperthyroidism.

Causes of clinical depression

The exact cause of a major depressive disorder or clinical depression is not known. However, there are many factors which can increase the risk of developing this condition. It has been observed that a combination of genes along with stress can affect the chemistry of the brain and therefore reduce the ability to maintain mood stability. Changes in hormones may also contribute to the development of MDD. High intake of alcohol and drug abuse or certain medical conditions and steroids may also trigger such type of depression.

How to identify if a person is under clinical depression?

Clinical depression is different from the feeling of sadness or stress. For example, it is very normal for a human being to feel depressed after a major disappointment at work or may have trouble sleeping in the case he had a break up in a relationship. In such scenarios people usually start feeling better after sharing or talking with a friend or family member. Whereas clinical depression is not the same, it involves changes which are noticeable and persist for two weeks or maybe longer. Let us imagine that a person has been sleeping for more than 10 hours every day and still feeling tired, complains of stomach problems, unable to cope with life and thinks that dying will solve all their problems. Sometimes the person doesn't want to spend time with family or friends and constantly feels irritable. Even if someone tries to reach out to them, the person gets more upset and moody. These are some of the experiences a person suffering from clinical depression will have.

Symptoms of clinical depression are:

A.   Feeling sad or depressed. In children and teenagers, a depressed mood can lead to constant irritability.

B.   There is no pleasure or reduced interest in all or most of their activities.

C.   Considerable amount of weight loss or weight gain without diet change.

D.   The desire to sleep more than normal or insomnia.

E.   Restlessness or slow behavior.

F.   Feeling tired or loss of energy.

G. A feeling of guilt or worthlessness.

H. Difficulty in decision making and concentrating.

I. Thoughts of committing suicide or about death.

Clinical depression can happen at any age, including children. According to the studies, major depressive disorder affects women more than men and it usually affects adults in the age group of 25-34 years old. The course of depression may vary while some may have recurrent episodes, others may experience bouts of depression spread over a long span of time. It has been observed that mental health conditions may often exist with major depressive disorder. Therefore it is advisable to consult the doctor in cases where natural remedies do not have positive results.

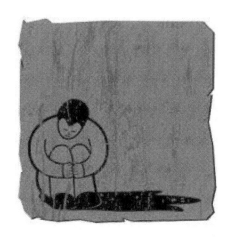

Treatment for Major Depressive Disorder

It is often treated with medication and psychological therapy. However, people who have severe MDD or have thoughts of harming themselves are advised to stay in the hospital under the care of health professionals.

The psychotherapy treatment involves meeting a therapist on a regular basis to discuss and talk about your condition. This process can help a person to adjust to stressful events, improve communication skills, replace negative feelings with positive ones, increase self-esteem and find better ways to cope with challenges.

However, it is also advised to adopt some lifestyle changes by keeping yourself healthy. An individual suffering from MDD should consider eating foods which are rich in omega-3 fatty acids like sprouts and fish. Also eating foods which are rich in Vitamin B such as whole grains and beans will help in staying fit. Avoid eating deep fried food and drinking alcohol which may have an adverse effect on the nervous system. Exercising outdoors in moderate sunlight can also make the person feel better.

Chapter VI: Other forms of depression

It is very normal to feel weak sometimes but if you are sad most of the time, and it affects your daily life, then you may be suffering from depression. This condition can be treated by either taking medicines, taking counseling from a therapist or even by doing some changes in your lifestyle. There are many forms of depression which may differ in their gravity from mild to severe depending on the person.

Types of acute depression along with their symptoms are mentioned below:

A)   **Persistent Depressive Disorder**- This type may persist for two years or more and is also known as 'dysthymia' in medical terms. As per the medical experts, genes may play a role but it is not necessarily true that most affected people have a family history. The following symptoms can help a person to get an idea if he is suffering from this type of depression –

1)   Change in appetite, either overeating or not being hungry leading to not eating.

2)   Sleeping for over 8 hours or insomnia.

3) Fatigue or lack of energy.

4) Feeling of low self-esteem.

5) Difficulty in concentrating.

6) Feeling of hopelessness.

B) **Bipolar disorder**- A person suffering from this kind of depression may have extreme mood swings. Bipolar disorder can also be termed as 'manic depression'. A person may feel the high energy with an 'up' mood and 'low' with depressive periods. Bipolar disorder may include the following warning signs:

1) Feeling elated for a prolonged period of time.

2) Getting agitated easily.

3) Talking very fast which is accompanied by racing thoughts.

4) Extremely impulsive.

5) Impaired judgment.

6) Overconfidence in your abilities.

7) Engaging in risky behavior such as gambling with life savings or splurging.

C) **Seasonal Affective Disorder**- It is usually experienced by people during the same time every year. People suffering from SAD have normal mental health but when there is a change of season for example, winter, when there is less sunlight and it is gloomy, many people suffer from seasonal affective order. It is also known as winter blues, winter depression, summer depression or seasonal depression. In most cases, the symptoms appear during early winter and go away during warm and sunny days of spring and summer. However, in the beginning, the symptoms are mild but they become more severe as the season progresses. Some SAD-specific symptoms are:

1. Irritability

2. Tiredness or feeling low on energy

3. Sleeping more than normal

4. Change in appetite which can lead to either weight gain or loss.

d) **Psychotic Depression**- Individuals with this disorder may suffer from symptoms such as hallucinations, delusions, and paranoia. People suffering from this type of depression may get angry without any evident reason or they may spend a lot of time alone in bed or staying away the whole night. They neglect their self-hygiene and may also talk less.

e)   **Postpartum Depression-** This condition strikes women in the first few months after childbirth. It can also happen after a miscarriage and a stillbirth. It can make one feel sorrowful, worthless and hopeless. The symptoms can last for a couple of months. This condition can occur due to changes in hormone level after pregnancy. A woman may have a greater chance of developing postpartum depression if she has suffered from depression before, doesn't have a good support system at home, if a baby is sick or any other stress in life.

f) **Pre-menstrual Dysphoric Disorder (PMDD)** – It is a condition where a woman has symptoms of severe depression like irritability and tension before menstruation. Women usually go through anxiety, mood swings, fatigue, food cravings, bloating, events of crying, muscle pains, and trouble sleeping. The reason for PMDD could be hormonal changes in the body. Apart from that, other factors such as thyroid disorder, being overweight, lack of physical activity and it may also happen if the woman has had a history of disease. If the symptoms become severe then they may interfere with daily routine. Some women even have thoughts about suicide and it is more likely to occur during the second half of their menstrual cycle.

g)   **Situational Depression**- According to mental health experts it is more of an adjustment disorder. It can occur in individuals as an aftermath of various traumatic changes in normal life such as the death of a loved one, divorce, losing a job, a break up in a relationship and severe illness. The symptoms can start within a couple of months following the event and they are similar to clinical depression. According to surveys done about 30% of youngsters and 10% of adults experience this condition at some point in their life and both men and women are affected equally with the symptoms. Depending on the individual, the symptoms can vary and include:

1.   Feeling of hopelessness

2.   Listlessness

3.   Sleeping difficulties

4.   Sadness

5.   Recurring bouts of crying

6.   Unfocussed anxiety

7. Loss of concentration

8. Worrying about anything and everything

9. Withdrawal from regular work, leisure activities, family and friends

10. In some cases, a person may even have suicidal thoughts.

h) **Atypical depression**- A person suffering from such depression may feel happy temporarily when there is a positive event which happens around him or her. With this disorder, a person might have symptoms such as a feeling of heaviness in arms and legs, increase in appetite, may feel over sensitive to any criticism, and hypersomnia (sleeping too much).

Acute depression is a serious medical condition which may have a severe impact on a person's ability to control his thoughts and behavior and in some cases it may also disrupt the capacity to perform day to day tasks. Treatment is crucial with this illness, since if left untreated, it may even lead to a suicidal attempt by the person.

Psychological counseling and medication are very effective for most people with depression. One may consult a doctor who can prescribe medications as per your condition. However, many people suffering from acute depression may also benefit from seeing a psychologist. Antidepressants are the most common medication prescribed by doctors.

Chapter VII: Co-existence of Anxiety and Depression

People often get confused between anxiety and depression and are usually not clear which one they suffer from.

What is anxiety?

Anxiety is a feeling of worry, nervousness or being uneasy about something which is uncertain. Typically, anxiety disorders are characterized by a sense of doubt or vulnerability about future events in life. Anxiety has various symptoms involving anxious thoughts, self-protective behaviors and sometimes unexplained physical sensations. Therefore, it is essential for a person to know if he is suffering from depression or anxiety. Individuals who suffer from depression doesn't show the same fear as people who suffer from anxiety. People who are depressed doesn't worry about the future, rather they believe that they already know what's going to happen and are somewhat sure that it's going to be bad.

There are several reasons why people get confused between anxiety and depression. One of the major reasons is that when they are prescribed antidepressants, and they search the web about the medication, they learn that the same medication is also prescribed to people with depression. Therefore, they start wondering if they are depressed. According to surveys done, 60% -70% of those who have depressive disorders also have anxiety, and almost half of those suffering from severe anxiety also have major symptoms of depression. Hence, we can say that anxiety and depression are just like the chicken and the egg story as to who came first. Over the years, clinical researchers have concluded that anxiety and depression are two faces of one disorder.

Under the following circumstances an anxiety disorder patient might need treatment for depression, they are:

a)   If the person is affected by stress and is left with no motivation or energy to overcome it. In such a case either behavioral methods or medication may be used to overcome depression.

b)   Secondly, if a person experiences severe depression before the anxiety disorder and it was not just a reaction to the difficulty imposed by anxiety disorders.

It is advisable that if one is confused about the symptoms of depression and anxiety than consulting a doctor or therapist would be a very good idea.

Why may anxiety lead to depression?

People suffering from anxiety disorders spend most of their life in an agitated state. After a long period of time it takes a huge toll emotionally, and then depression sets in. According to the Anxiety and Depression Association of America, there is no conclusive justification as to why anxiety and depression co-exist so often.

It has been observed that anxiety disorders are much more than worrying and nervousness. Many people think that their thoughts are irrational but they still are not able to stop themselves. There are a few symptoms which have been summarized below to give a better understanding of a person who may be suffering from both anxiety and depression-

a) Constant irrational worrying

b) Physical effects like headaches, fatigue, hot flashes, sweating, rapid heartbeat, difficulty in breathing and abdominal pain.

c) Insomnia

d) Change in their eating pattern

e) Trouble in memorizing things and concentration

f) Constant feeling of worthlessness

g) Loss of interest in hobbies

h) Feeling cranky and irritable

i) Unable to relax

j) Sometimes even panic attacks

Apart from these generalized symptoms there are some warning signs which can be noticed by the loved ones who are close to the person suffering from both anxiety and depression-

a) Such people lose interest in daily self-care and personal hygiene

b) They have extreme mood swings

c) Sometimes they may even get violent, aggressive or may even abusive

d) They may appear confused most of the time or may hallucinate things

e) Talking about death or committing suicide.

The Recovery path

Both depression and anxiety should be treated together. Some of the common treatment strategies include:

A) **Cognitive behavioral therapy or CBT**- This therapy teaches people how to manage their anxiety and depression symptoms by figuring out the cause for them. People learn how to control their emotions.

B) **Medication**- the therapist or the doctor may advise certain medicines according to the condition of the individual.

C) **Exercise**- It is a natural way of treating both anxiety and depression. While exercising, the body releases chemicals that make you feel good and relax. Like taking a walk may help to reduce the symptoms.

D) **Relaxing**- Relaxation techniques such as meditation can ease the symptoms of both anxiety and depression.

Chapter VIII: Remedies to treat acute depression

After getting insight into the types of depression, let us look at some remedial measures which can be used in curing the person suffering from severe depression.

a) Persistent Depressive Disorder (Dysthymia)

The treatment approach which is recommended by the doctors depends on upon the severity of the symptoms, personal preferences and desire and willingness of the person. Psychotherapy is typically recommended for children and adolescents who are suffering from this type of disorder. Apart from medications, there are some natural remedies which can be easily adapted to treat the patient.

1.   The first and foremost step is to be aware of the symptoms and look out for any warning signs.

2.   Stay healthy by eating a proper diet and get sufficient sleep.

3.   Involve yourself in some activities like jogging, running, swimming, gardening or any other activity which you enjoy doing.

4. Avoid alcohol since in long term it worsens the depression.

5. Set goals for yourself and stay motivated and focused on achieving them so that you have something to look forward.

6. Plan your day well and keep yourself busy with daily chores.

7. Stay connected with friends and family.

8. Participate in social activities.

9. Avoid making any decisions when you are feeling depressed since you may not be able to think clearly.

10. Lastly, learn ways to relax and manage your stress.

b) **Bipolar Disorder**

There are a few home remedies which can be used to treat bipolar disorder.

1. Diet- Although there is no particular bipolar diet, it is important to make sensible dietary choices that will help you to maintain a healthy weight and stay fit. One should try and avoid red meat, saturated fats, and carbohydrates. Eat balanced nutrient rich foods like

fresh fruits, legumes, green vegetables, whole grains, soy products, fish, nuts, etc. Always keep a check on calorie intake and do regular exercise.

2.   Well- Being- The mood swings under bipolar disorder can be incredibly destructive. They can isolate the person from friends and family. Always keep lines of communication with near and dear ones open, talk to them and discuss with them what you feel. Try to hear what they have to say and apologize in case you've hurt them.

c) **Seasonal Affective Disorder**

1.   People may feel gloomy and depressed as days are short in winter. Try and brighten up your home by decorating it in such a way that the maximum natural light comes into the house. Keep your curtains and blinds open.

2.   On sunny winter days, take a walk outdoors.

3.   Try and plan a vacation to a warmer place.

4.   Join a health club or gym.

d) **Psychotic Depression**

Usually, psychotic depression patients are closely monitored by professionals, and they may also give medications to stabilize the patient's mood. Apart from that, there are certain natural cures for this type of depression.

1.   Green Cardamom- Intake of green cardamoms can control psychotic depression to an extent. These seeds have excellent healing properties for the nervous system in human body. The best way to take it is to mix the cardamom powder in tea with a small amount of sugar.

2.   Avoid alcohol and drugs- These directly affect the nervous system and hence should be prevented.

3.   Regular exercise -Keep your body fit by doing some basic exercises.

4.   One should try and develop an interest or a hobby so as to keep the brain occupied.

5.   Fish is rich in Omega3 and eating fish on a regular basis for at least three months will help in stabilizing the mind and will also contribute to improving the mental condition.

E) **Postpartum Depression**

This type of depression can be treated with counseling and medication but there are a few basic natural remedies which one can follow:

1. Get rest- New parents should ensure that their sleep cycle is maintained. In case you have a support system at home like in-laws they can help you with the baby. Avoid using over the counter sleep aids.

2. Eat healthy- A proper nutritious diet can make a huge difference in regulating hormones in the body since during the times of stress or change body uses excess nutrients. One should eat a lot of green leafy vegetables, whole grains, and fruits to ensure a balanced intake of proteins, vitamins and minerals.

3. Reduce stress by maintaining a proper schedule. One can try to cut down family or social outings. Practice some relaxation exercises like yoga, meditation or acupressure.

4. Take time for self-grooming and care

5.   Listen to some music, spend time with friends, laugh and stay happy.

6.   Sometimes expressing your thoughts by writing may also help.

F) **Pre-menstrual Dysphoric Disorder (PMDD)**

Some remedies are commonly used for PMDD symptoms apart from vitamin supplements which your doctor may advise.

1.   Do regular exercise, at least 30 minutes in a day.

2.   Avoid intake of caffeine, sugar and alcohol.

3.   Engage yourself in physical activities, meditation, yoga or even aerobics.

4.   Eat healthy food which should include whole grains, green vegetables, and fruits.

5.   One should also reduce the quantity of salt used in food.

g) Situational Depression

This type of depression is curable and in most of the cases the person gets relief in a short period of time. You need to follow a healthy lifestyle which includes eating a proper diet, reducing alcohol consumption, avoiding late sleeping and exercising regularly.

h) Atypical depression

Be aware of your situation so that you can pay attention to the warning signs. You should take care of yourself by staying healthy, physically active by getting involved in any types of sports activity and avoid alcohol and drugs.

Therefore, we can conclude that a person needs to maintain a healthy lifestyle and stay happy to overcome any depression. Given below are few examples of some famous celebrities who suffered from depression and how they came out of it. We are writing it to ensure that our readers know that it is curable and not a disease with which you have for the rest of your life.

1. A very popular figure in the Indian music industry was suffering from bipolar disorder. He was fighting extreme emotions and was unable to keep control over it. He changed doctors four times and no medication was helping him. He had cut himself from friends and family and didn't care about his looks. He got his courage from his mother and his self-belief got him out of this suffering.

2. Recently a famous actress came out in the media and said that she was suffering from depression at the time when she was establishing herself in the entertainment industry. She used to experience a nagging feeling, shallow breath and lack of concentration. She was resistant to take up any treatment and then she heard about her friend's death due to anxiety and depression. This changed her mind and she agreed to go through counseling and medication which finally brought her out of her depression.

3. A very famous Hollywood star suffered from depression in his early days of his acting career. He used to take drugs and was cut off from the outside world. After he had taken a trip to Casablanca, he saw extreme poverty which he had never witnessed before.

This changed his mind and helped him come out of his depression.

4.   Another famous American actress fell into depression in the year 2008 after her mother had passed away. She felt that she was going to a dark place and was unable to get up in the morning. She then signed up for a movie and did a regular physical activity to come out of her depression successfully.

Depression doesn't discriminate and it can happen to anyone at any time during their life. Celebrities live a lavish, luxurious and elegant life, and it seems that they have it all but they are human too. So one can take inspiration from them as to how they came out of their depression. Most of them are doing their bit to spread awareness about mental health. According to the World Health Organization, depression was ranked as the third leading disease in 2004 and may move into a first place by 2030.

Chapter IX: How to help a person suffering from depression and setting boundaries

Now that we understand severe forms of depression, their symptoms and treatment, we should also know that individuals who take care of depressed individuals also have a task in hand. People suffering from depression often resist seeking help. Prejudices about mental illness may stop a person from getting a diagnosis and so avoids the treatment. Whereas, many other patients simply fail to understand or see that they are not acting like themselves. That's where the role of a loved one comes in. It is upon the people who are closest to the depressed person to urge them gently but firmly to seek help.

Going into depression isn't anybody's fault and neither is it by choice, it is just a condition suffered by an individual. A caregiver must understand the following:

a. In case the depressed person is agitated, restless or abusive one must know that these attacks are not personal.

b. Keep yourself involved in the treatment plan of your loved one, whether it is medication, psychotherapy or both. They will need your constant support and encouragement. You should be willing to listen and also be vigilant in case of acute cases since some people get suicidal thoughts.

c. Make sure that your loved one is eating and sleeping properly.

d. It is very normal that if depression strikes a loved one the partner or spouse may focus all his or her energy in helping the patient. It is essential for the caregiver to take care of themselves, get additional support from extended family or friends in case the situation is out of control but don't get burdened and stressed out.

e. Lastly, keep in mind to approach your loved one who is suffering gently with compassion and understanding and not judgment.

Setting boundaries with a depressed person

When you are taking care of someone who is suffering from depression, it is important to discuss and talk about the behaviors that are dangerous or unacceptable. Few guidelines which can be considered are:

a. **Adhere to the treatment plan**- Tell the person that you care about them but it is not possible for you to do that alone and explain that how seeking professional help would benefit him or her. Insist they attend all sessions or going for appointments with a health professional.

b. **Stand up to abuse**- Firmly explain to the person that such behavior is entirely unacceptable to you and he or she should avoid it entirely.

c. **Live with healthy habits**- Encourage the person to channel his or her energy into some constructive activities such as exercising or hobbies. Make sure that they are eating healthy food.

Some frequently asked questions on depression

1.   Why is depression more common in women than men?

Ans: Yes, depression is more common in women than men. Surveys have revealed that about 20% of women have at least one episode of depression in their lifetime since biological, hormonal and psychological factors unique to women can be linked to high depression rates. However, it has been found that before adolescence both girls and boys suffer from depression at the same frequency but once they pass that stage of life girls have more chances of falling into depression.

2.   Do elderly people suffer from depression?

Ans: Yes, such conditions can arise anytime during a person's life and for people who experience it later in life, some factors like changes in the body or the functioning of the brain may have a role to play. For e.g. with age, blood vessels become less flexible and may prevent normal blood flow to the brain. If this occurs, then an elderly person with no family history of depression may develop the condition.

3. Is depression hereditary?

Ans: As we grow up we learn different attributes of life from people close to us so if we see it from that point of view, depression as a way of behaving or seeing things it can be passed on.

4. Can children also fall into depression?

Ans: Yes, children can go into depression and causes can be similar to any adult. Children who suffer from depression may experience a change in their behavior which can be persistent and upset their healthy lifestyle. They may lose interest in school and make them cut their ties from friends.

5. Why is there an increase in the many people suffering from mental health issues?

Ans: This could be due to stresses of modern day and our fast paced life. This could also be due to the increasing awareness about the condition.

6. Is lack of sleep a cause of depression?

Ans: No, lack of sleep is not the only reason which can make a person go into depression but it may play a role in intensifying the problem.

7. Why does one feel depressed even if everything around them is fine?

Ans: A person may have a happy and healthy life with supportive family, good job and financial security but may still feel unsatisfied and unhappy. Irrespective of the external factors, it is the internal factors that are more important. A person should be able to experience appropriate emotional satisfaction from his surroundings. For e.g. if you achieve something great at work, you think 'Oh! Anybody can do that', 'it is not something great' then it can lead to the lack of self-confidence and meaning in life.

8. If someone has suffered from depression once, is it likely that he will become depressed again?

Ans: A person who has experienced depression once does put him or her at a higher risk of the same condition again. Therefore getting proper treatment at the appropriate time is essential for recovery and also to prevent any future episodes.

9. Can menopause trigger depression?

Ans: As menopause sets in the lifecycle of a woman, the possibility increases for some of them to experience depression due to the fall in hormone levels which affect the brain.

10. How can people help themselves during depression?

Ans: If one wants to do self-help then the first and most important thing is to understand oneself. Do things that keep you occupied, regulate your sleep patterns, eat healthy and most importantly do not think too much.

Conclusion

Everybody goes through ups and downs in their life but life goes on. We need to be in control of ourselves to overcome that overwhelming feeling that the whole world is conspiring against us or bad things happen to just us. One has to strive to get over the sadness, negativity and feeling of hopelessness in life. We should stay happy and enjoy the good things around us, cherish the moments of life with your loved ones.

To sum it up, beating depression is not about moving away from the things happening around us rather it is how we respond to life events whether good or bad.

Thank you again for getting this book and for taking that step towards getting away from depression and being happy.

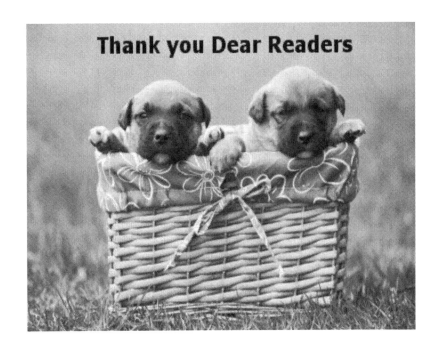

We hope this book was able to help you understand depression, identify it and load you with techniques not just to fight it but also to stay away from it forever.

Your next steps – what should they be:

Step one - Take action right away. Implement these techniques as soon as you can. The best way is to incorporate two techniques every day which means by the end of two months you would have tried all of them.

Even if you manage to absorb just 10% of the above mentioned techniques into your daily routine and life-style, you will see a huge positive shift in your life.

We really hope that you get maximum benefit out of this book.

Step two - Help people who are facing similar issues of depression, stress and anxiety.

We would like to take this book to as many people as possible and help them deal with challenges in life by giving them these simple techniques to life-long happiness.

Please assist us in this effort.

Kindly post a review for this book and let others know how you liked it.

Below is the link which will take you to the review section directly.

http://amzn.to/1YoqDoQ

Your feedback is valuable to us!

Get your Double Bonus –

Absolutely FREE

As a thank you for your review and for buying this book, we would like to give you a couple of FREE gifts.

Please go to the link below to download for FREE – **Using Affirmations for Success.**

http://bit.ly/1NUyyjA

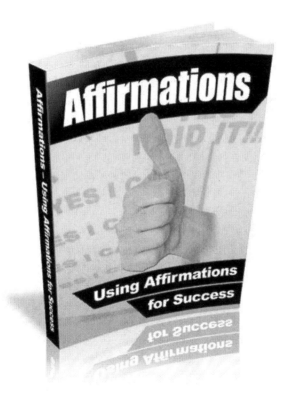

Please go to the link below and download for FREE –

100 Interview Tips to prepare you for that all important meeting of your life and help you secure your dream job.

http://bit.ly/25shcCm

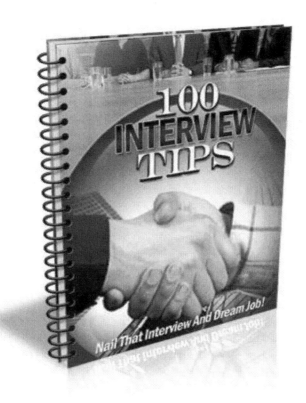

We hope you liked your FREE gifts.

Please do visit us on our website

www.ShiningUniverseEnergy.com

We would love to see you there!

Like us on **Facebook**

https://www.facebook.com/shininguniverseenergy

Follow us on **Twitter @ShiningUE**

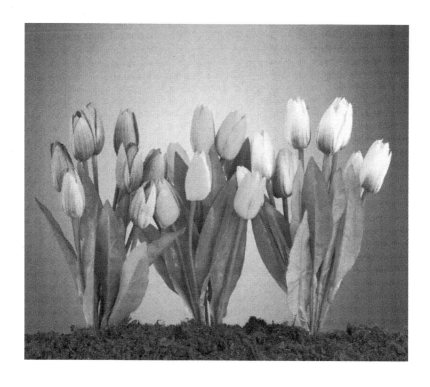

Please check our other book **'Brain: 51 Powerful Ways to Improve Brain Power, Enhance Memory, Intelligence and Concentration NATURALLY'**

This is available world-wide on all bookstore websites. Here is the link to get this book http://lrd.to/brain

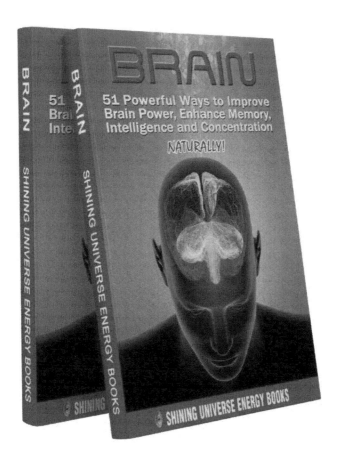

Printed in Great Britain
by Amazon